FUEL YOUR BODY RIGHT

FINDING THE PERFECT PORTION SIZE FOR OPTIMAL HEALTH

VIKRAM GOPAL

CONTENTS

PREFACE

Portion control is an essential aspect of maintaining good health. By following the tips discussed in this article, you can find the perfect portion size for optimal health. Remember that portion control is not about depriving yourself of your favorite foods, but rather learning how to eat in moderation and make smart food choices. By practicing portion control, you can achieve a balanced diet, maintain a healthy weight, and reduce your risk of developing various health problems.

I am happy to present my readers this unique book to help them achieve their health goals.

Vikram Gopal
20th March 2023

INTRODUCTION

Eating the right amount of food is essential for maintaining good health. Portion control plays a crucial role in achieving a balanced diet and maintaining a healthy weight. Consuming too much or too little food can have negative impacts on our health. In this article, we will discuss the importance of portion control and provide tips on how to find the perfect portion size for optimal health.

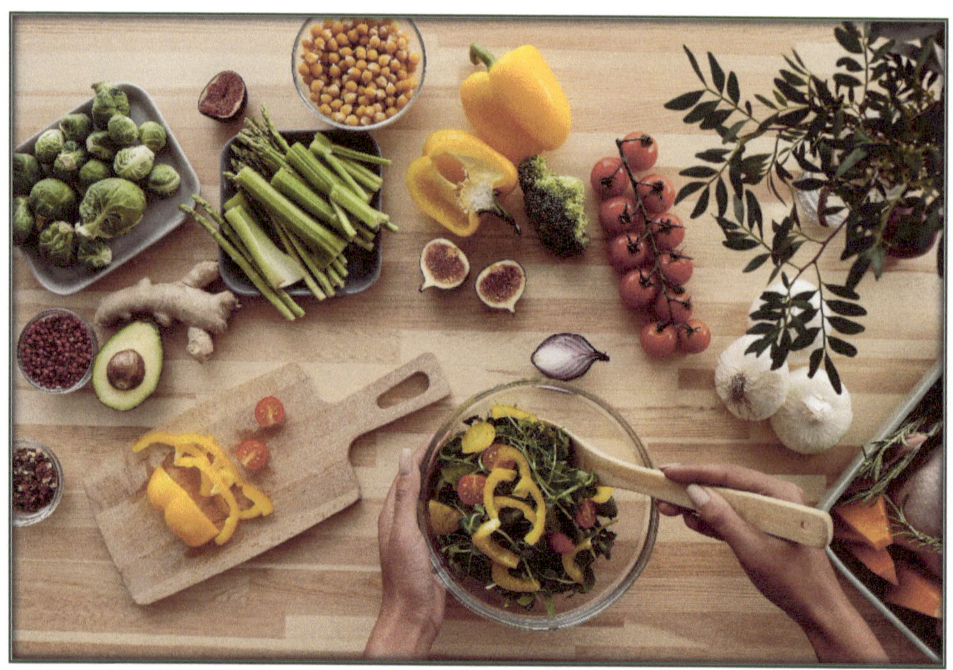

The Importance of Portion Control:

Portion control is the practice of eating a specific amount of food. It is not about depriving yourself of your favorite foods or following a strict diet plan. Instead, it is about learning how to eat in moderation and make smart food choices. Eating too much food can lead to weight gain and obesity, which increases the risk of developing various health problems such as diabetes, heart disease, and cancer. On the other hand, consuming too little food can result in malnutrition, which can lead to various deficiencies, weakness, and other health problems.

Tips for Finding the Perfect Portion Size:

1. Use Measuring Cups and Spoons: Measuring cups and spoons are a great tool for controlling portion sizes. You can use them to measure out the recommended serving size for different food groups, such as grains, fruits, vegetables, and protein.
2. Learn to Estimate Portion Sizes: If you do not have measuring cups and spoons, you can still estimate portion sizes by using your hand as a guide. For example, a serving of protein should be the size of your palm, while a serving of grains should be the size of your fist.
3. Use Smaller Plates: Using smaller plates can help you control your portion sizes. When you use a large plate, you tend to fill it up, which can lead to overeating. However, when you use a smaller plate, you will naturally eat less.
4. Avoid Eating Straight Out of the Bag or Box: When you eat straight out of the bag or box, it is easy to lose track of how

much you are eating. Instead, portion out your food onto a plate or bowl before eating.

5. Slow Down and Enjoy Your Food: Eating slowly and savoring each bite can help you feel more satisfied with smaller portions. When you eat too quickly, you are more likely to overeat because your brain does not have enough time to register that you are full.

6. Listen to Your Body: Pay attention to your body's hunger and fullness signals. Eat when you are hungry and stop when you are full. Do not eat just because there is food in front of you or because it is a certain time of day.

USE MEASURING CUPS AND SPOONS

Using measuring cups and spoons is an effective way to control portion sizes because it allows you to accurately measure the recommended serving size for different food groups. When you are aware of how much food you are consuming, it becomes easier to manage your calorie intake and achieve a balanced diet.

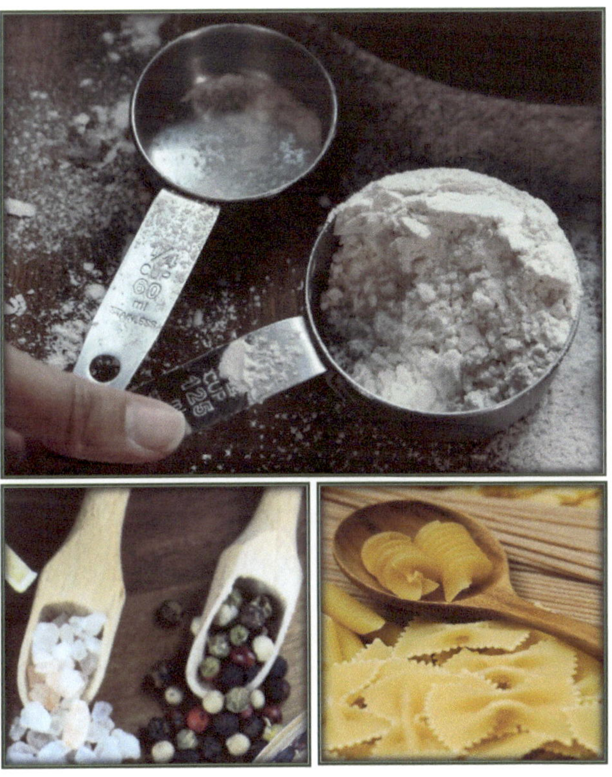

For example, a serving of grains is typically one-half cup of cooked rice or pasta, which is equivalent to about the size of your fist. However, it can be challenging to determine the correct serving size by simply eyeballing it. By using a measuring cup, you can be sure that you are consuming the appropriate amount.

Similarly, a serving of protein, such as chicken or fish, is typically three ounces, or about the size of the palm of your hand. Measuring out three ounces with a kitchen scale or using a measuring cup can ensure that you are not over or under-eating.

Fruits and vegetables also have specific serving sizes that can be easily measured using measuring cups and spoons. For example, one serving of fruit is typically one medium-sized piece, such as an apple or a banana, or one-half cup of chopped fruit. For vegetables, one serving is typically one-half cup of cooked or raw vegetables.

In addition to controlling portion sizes, using measuring cups and spoons can also help you be more mindful of your food choices. When you measure out your food, you are more likely to pay close attention to the type of food and how much you are consuming. This can help you make better food choices and prevent excessive eating.

In summary, using measuring cups and spoons is a simple but effective way to control portion sizes and ensure that you are consuming the appropriate amount of food. By measuring out your food, you can manage your calorie intake, achieve a balanced diet, and prevent overeating.

LEARN TO ESTIMATE PORTION SIZES

Learning to estimate portion sizes is an essential skill for managing your calorie intake and achieving a balanced diet. It is particularly useful when you don't have access to measuring cups and spoons. One helpful tip is to use your hand as a guide to estimate portion sizes for different food groups.

For example, a serving of protein, such as chicken, beef, or fish, should be roughly the size of your palm. This estimate provides a quick and easy way to gauge how much protein you should be consuming in each meal. If you are having a larger meal, such as a dinner, you may need to have two servings of protein.

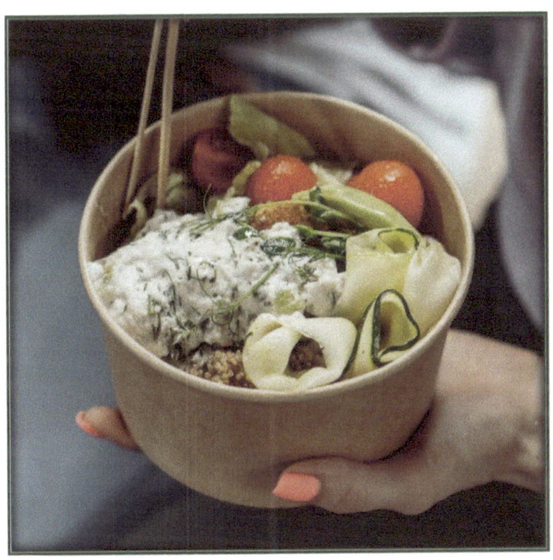

A serving of grains, such as rice, pasta, or quinoa, should be about the size of your fist. This estimate can help you control your portion sizes and ensure that you are not overeating. If you are having a sandwich, a serving of grains would be equivalent to one slice of bread.

For vegetables, a serving size is usually one-half cup of cooked or raw vegetables. To estimate this portion size, you can use your hand as a guide by forming a fist and then opening your hand. The amount of vegetables that can fit in your hand should be about one-half cup.

For fruits, one serving is usually one medium-sized piece, such as an apple or a banana. To estimate this portion size, you can use your hand again by forming a fist. The size of your fist should be similar to that of a medium-sized piece of fruit.

It is important to note that these portion size estimates are general guidelines and may vary depending on your individual needs and goals. They can, however, serve as a helpful starting point for managing your calorie intake and achieving a balanced diet.

In summary, learning to estimate portion sizes using your hand as a guide is an effective way to manage your calorie intake and achieve a balanced diet, especially when you don't have access to measuring cups and spoons. By using these estimates, you can control your portion sizes and ensure that you are consuming the appropriate amount of food for your body's needs.

USE SMALLER PLATES

Using smaller plates is a simple yet effective way to control your portion sizes and prevent overeating. When you use a large plate, it is easy to fill it up with more food than your body needs. However, when you use a smaller plate, you can create the illusion of a full plate without consuming too much food.

Research has shown that people tend to eat more when they are presented with larger portions of food. This phenomenon is known as the "portion size effect" and can lead to overeating and weight gain over time. By using smaller plates, you can trick

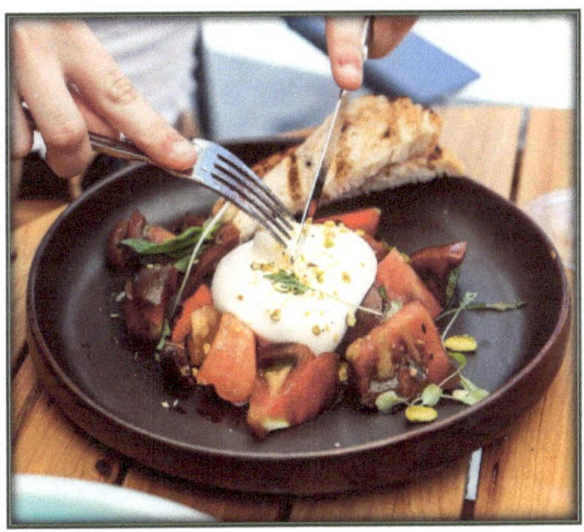

your mind into thinking that you are consuming a full meal, even if the actual amount of food is smaller.

In addition, using smaller plates can help you develop better eating habits over time. When you consistently use smaller plates, you may find that you become more aware of your portion sizes and begin to naturally consume less food. This can lead to long-term weight management and better overall health.

It is essential to note that using smaller plates alone is not a solution for unhealthy eating habits. It is crucial to combine this approach with other healthy habits such as choosing nutritious foods, practicing mindful eating, and incorporating regular exercise into your routine.

In summary, using smaller plates is a simple but effective way to control your portion sizes and prevent overeating. By creating the illusion of a full plate with less food, you can trick your mind into consuming fewer calories. Over time, using smaller plates can help you develop better eating habits and maintain a healthy weight.

AVOID EATING STRAIGHT OUT OF THE BAG OR BOX

Avoiding eating straight out of the bag or box is an essential step to controlling your portion sizes and preventing overeating. When you eat directly from a container, it is easy to lose track of how much you are consuming. Before you know it, you may have eaten far more than you intended.

Portioning out your food onto a plate or bowl before eating helps you to become more aware of your food choices and the amount you are eating. It allows you to visualize your portion size and control your intake. Portioning also makes it easier to track your food intake and adjust your portion sizes to meet your dietary goals.

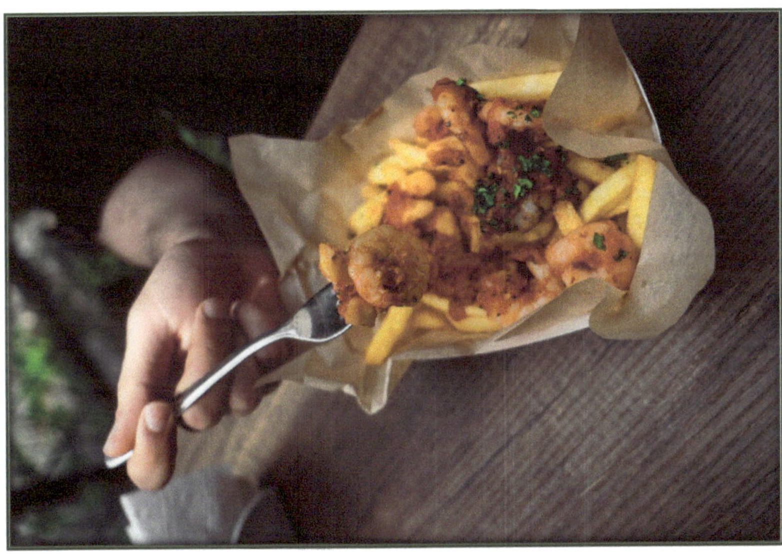

Another advantage of portioning out your food is that it can help you enjoy your food more fully. When you eat directly from the bag or box, you may not pay as much attention to your food, and you may not fully savor the taste and texture. By portioning your food, you create a more mindful eating experience that allows you to enjoy each bite.

One way to make portioning easier is to invest in small bowls or plates. These can be used to control the amount of food you consume in each meal, and they provide a clear visual cue for how much food you should eat. You can also use measuring cups or spoons to ensure that you are consuming the recommended serving size of different food groups.

In summary, avoiding eating straight out of the bag or box is a simple yet effective way to control your portion sizes and prevent overeating. By portioning out your food onto a plate or bowl, you become more aware of your food choices, and you can better control your calorie intake. This can help you develop healthy eating habits and maintain a healthy weight over time.

SLOW DOWN AND ENJOY YOUR FOOD

Slowing down and savoring your food is an essential strategy to control your portion sizes and prevent overeating. When you eat too quickly, your brain does not have enough time to register the signals that indicate fullness. This can lead to overeating and consuming more calories than your body needs.

Eating slowly and mindfully, on the other hand, can help you become more aware of your food choices and the amount you are consuming. It allows you to fully experience the taste and texture of your food, which can enhance your enjoyment of the meal. Moreover, by taking the time to chew your food properly and savor each bite, you give your brain more time to receive signals of fullness and satisfaction.

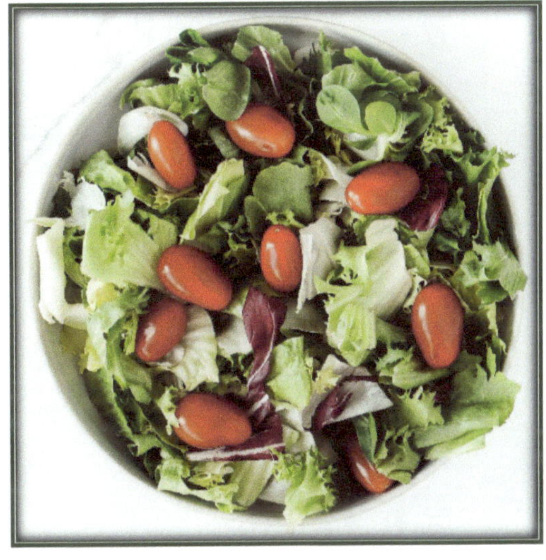

One way to practice mindful eating is to put down your utensils between each bite and take the time to savor the food. You can also try to identify the different flavors and textures in your meal, such as the sweetness of fruit or the crunch of vegetables. By taking the time to focus on your food, you can better appreciate the flavors and feel more satisfied with smaller portions.

Another way to slow down your eating is to eliminate distractions while you eat. Avoid eating in front of the television or computer, as these activities can divert your attention from your food and lead to mindless eating. Instead, try to eat in a calm and relaxing environment, such as at a table with friends or family.

In summary, slowing down and enjoying your food is a crucial strategy to control your portion sizes and prevent overeating. By taking the time to savor your food and focus on your meal, you can better regulate your appetite and feel more satisfied with smaller portions. Practicing mindful eating and eliminating distractions during meals can help you develop healthy eating habits and maintain a healthy weight over time

LISTEN TO YOUR BODY

Listening to your body's hunger and fullness signal is a crucial aspect of controlling your portion sizes and preventing overeating. Eating only when you are hungry and stopping when you are full can help you develop healthy eating habits and maintain a healthy weight.

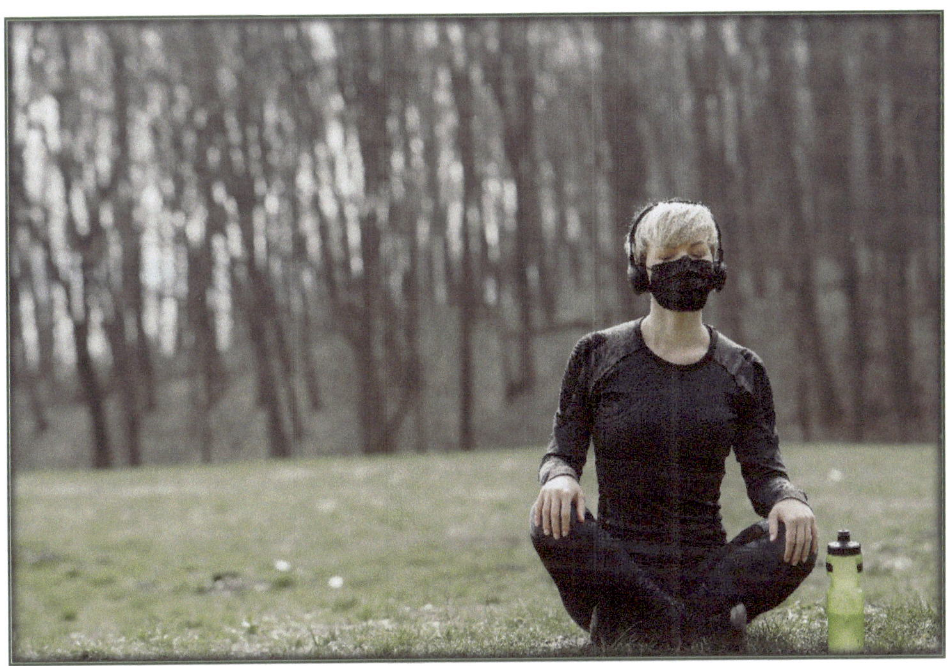

One of the best ways to listen to your body is to pay attention to your hunger and fullness signals. Hunger cues can include feelings of emptiness or grumbling in your stomach, while fullness cues can include feelings of satisfaction and contentment. Eating only when you are hungry and stopping when you are full can help you avoid overeating and consuming more calories than your body needs.

Another way to listen to your body is to avoid eating just because there is food in front of you or because it is a certain time of day. Eating out of boredom or habit can lead to mindless eating and consuming more calories than your body needs. Instead, try to tune into your body's needs and eat only when you are hungry and need fuel.

Moreover, it is also essential to slow down and pay attention to your body while you eat. Take the time to savor each bite and listen to your body's signals of fullness. If you find yourself feeling full or satisfied before finishing your meal, stop eating and save the rest for later.

It is also important to note that everyone's hunger and fullness signals are different. What works for one person may not work for another. Therefore, it is crucial to develop a personalized approach to listening to your body and determining when to eat and when to stop.

In summary, listening to your body's hunger and fullness signal is an essential strategy for controlling your portion sizes and preventing overeating. Eating only when you are hungry and stopping when you are full can help you develop healthy eating habits and maintain a healthy weight. By paying attention to your body's needs and signals, you can develop a personalized approach to eating that works best for you

IMPORTANT POINTS TO BE CONSIDERED

Here are some key points to consider for optimal health based on "Fuel Your Body Right: Finding the Perfect Portion Size":

1. Portion control: It is important to be mindful of how much you eat at each meal. Eating too much can lead to weight gain and other health problems. Aim to eat smaller, more frequent meals throughout the day to keep your energy levels up.

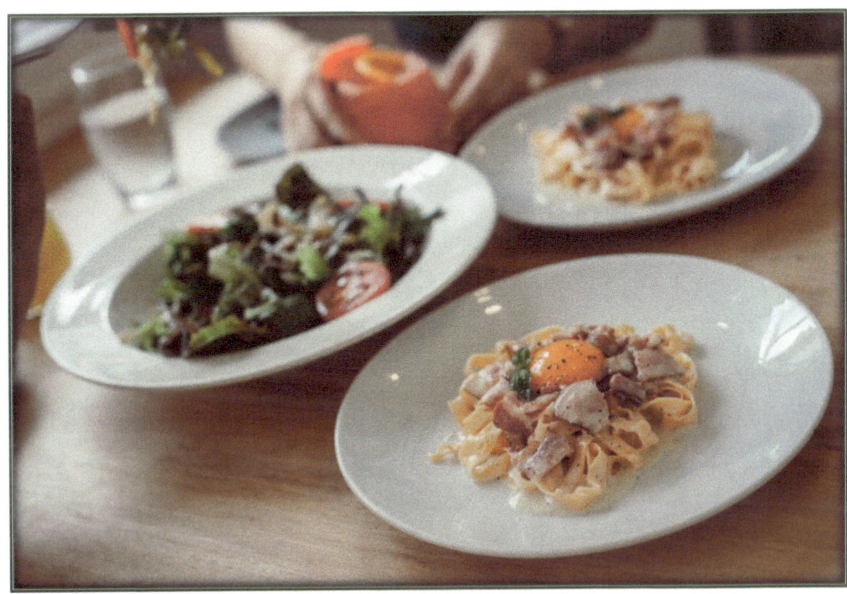

2. Balanced meals: Ensure that your meals are balanced with a variety of nutrients, including carbohydrates, protein, and

healthy fats. This will help you feel fuller for longer and prevent cravings.

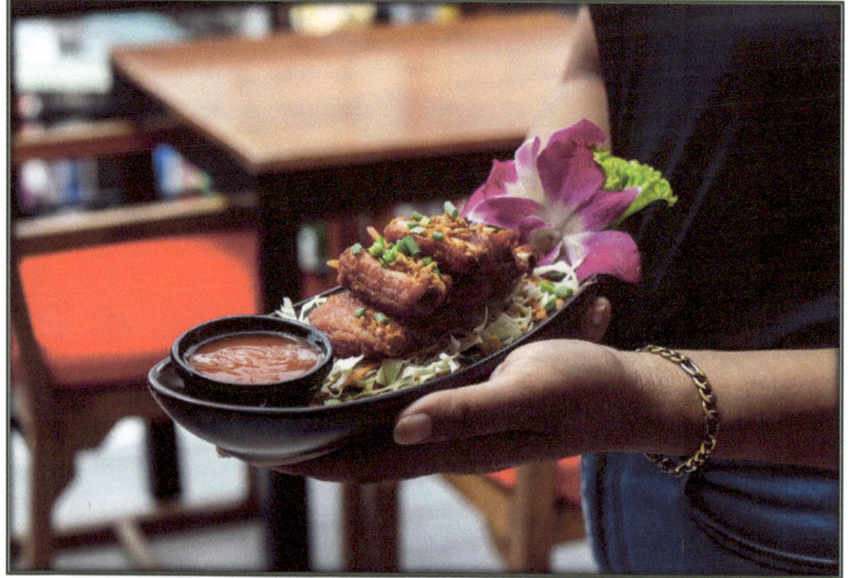

3. Quality of food: Choose high-quality, nutrient-dense foods that provide your body with the fuel it needs. Avoid processed foods and limit your intake of sugar and unhealthy fats.

4. Listen to your body: It's important to be in tune with your body's hunger and fullness signals. Stop eating once you feel content rather than overly stuffed, and take note of these signals to avoid overeating and maintain appropriate portion sizes. This approach will help you stay mindful and prevent overindulgence.

5. Exercise: Regular exercise is an important component of a healthy lifestyle. It helps you maintain a healthy weight, improves your overall health, and boosts your mood.

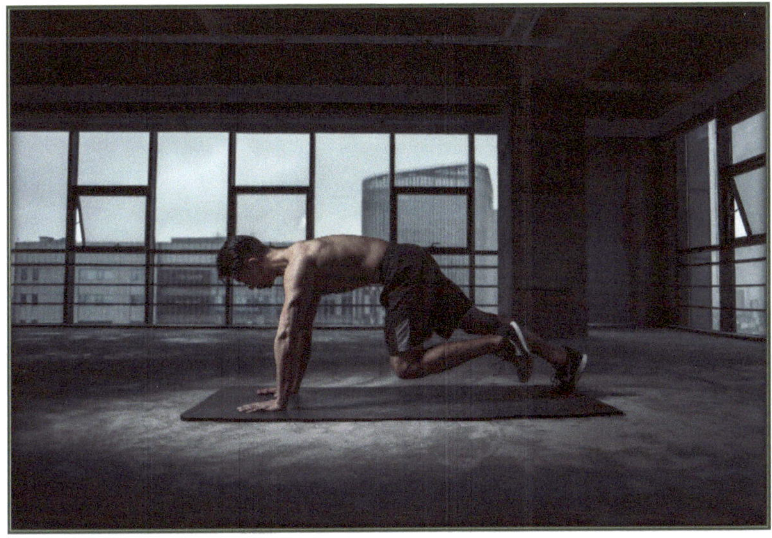

6. Mindful eating: Take the time to enjoy your food and eat without distractions. This can help you tune in to your body's hunger and fullness signals and prevent overeating.

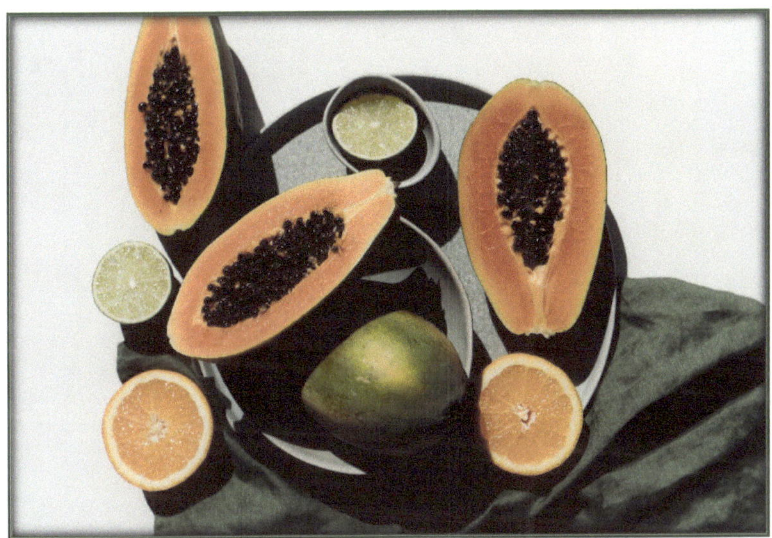

7. Hydration: Drinking enough water is essential for good health. Aim to drink at least eight glasses of water per day to stay hydrated and help your body function properly.

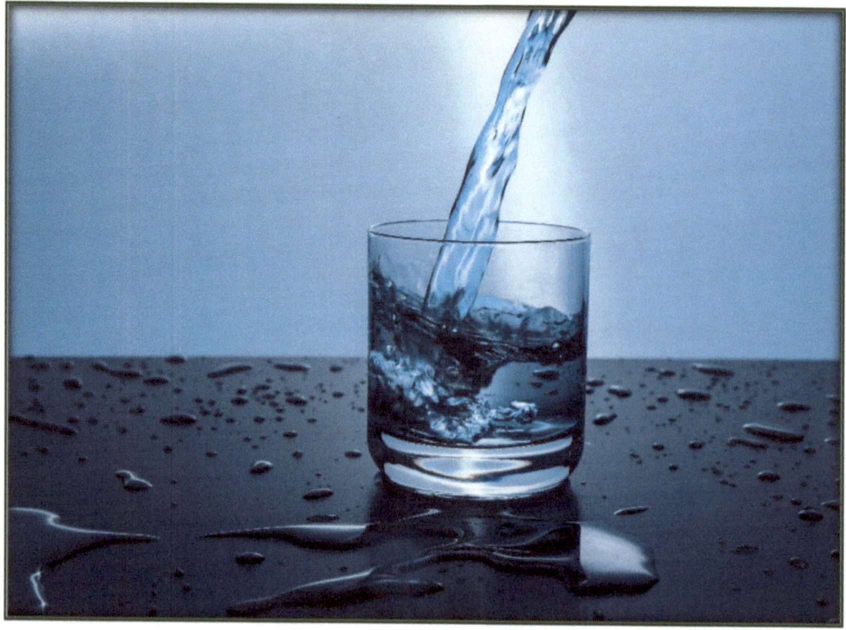

By following these key points, you can fuel your body right and find the perfect portion size for optimal health.

CONCLUSION

In conclusion, portion control is a vital aspect of maintaining a healthy diet and achieving optimal health. By understanding the recommended serving sizes for different food groups and using tools such as measuring cups, spoons, and smaller plates, you can control your portions and avoid overeating.

It is also important to remember to slow down and savor your food, listen to your body's hunger and fullness responses, and avoid eating straight out of the bag or box. By developing a personalized approach to portion control, you can maintain a healthy weight and reduce your risk of chronic diseases such as obesity, type 2 diabetes, and heart disease.

In addition to portion control, it is essential to focus on consuming a balanced diet that includes a variety of nutrient-dense foods such as variety of fruits, colorful vegetables, different type of whole grains, lean proteins, and healthy fats. By fueling your body with the right nutrients and controlling your portions, you can optimize your health and wellbeing.

However, it is important to remember that achieving optimal health is a journey, not a destination. It takes time, effort, and dedication to develop healthy habits and maintain them over time. Therefore, it is crucial to be patient, stay committed to your goals, and seek support from friends, family, or a healthcare professional if needed.

In summary, portion control is a crucial component of a healthy diet and can help you achieve optimal health. By implementing the tips and strategies outlined in this article, you can develop a personalized approach to portion control and fuel your body right. Remember to focus on consuming a balanced diet, listen to your body, and stay committed to your goals. With time and effort, you can achieve optimal health and wellbeing.